A WALKING

A SURVIVOR'S JOURNEY

TALKING

THROUGH LIVER FAILURE & FAITH

MIRACLE

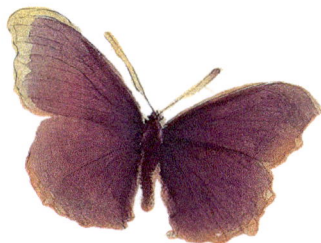

YVONNE WEAVER

KP PUBLISHING COMPANY

ISBN: 978-1-960001-96-2 (Hardcover)
ISBN: 978-1-960001-92-4 (Paperback)
ISBN: 978-1-960001-93-1 (eBook)

Library of Congress Control Number: Pending

Editor: Manuscript Mender
Cover Design: Juan Roberts, Creative Lunacy
Literary Director: Sandra Slayton James

Published by:

KP Publishing Company
Publisher of Fiction, Nonfiction & Children's Books
Las Vegas, NV 89117
www.kp-pub.com

Printed in the United States of America

DEDICATION

I lovingly dedicate this book to my maternal grandmother, Marina Lloyd, and my paternal grandmother, Mother Emma Schley, women whose faithful prayers covered my life long before I understood their power.

They did more than speak to me about Christ; they lived Him before me. Through their love, discipline, sacrifice, and unwavering faith, they modeled the grace and truth of lives fully surrendered to God. Their legacy reflects the wisdom of Proverbs 22:6:

> *"Train up a child in the way he should go, and when he is old, he will not depart from it."*

Because they prayed, believed, and walked by faith, I stand today as living evidence that *"the effectual fervent prayer of a righteous woman availeth much"* (James 5:16).

I have survived chronic illness because of the legacy of strength, courage, and healing that runs through our veins.

I stand on the shoulders of Marina Lloyd and Mother Emma Schley, and I walk forward strengthened by their faith, covered by their prayers, and sustained by the generations of healing they set in motion.

"I shall not die, but live,
And declare the works of the Lord."
Psalm 118:17 (NKJV)

CONTENTS

"But those who hope in the Lord
will renew their strength.
They will soar on wings like eagles;
they will run and not grow weary,
they will walk and not be faint."
Isaiah 40:31 (NIV)

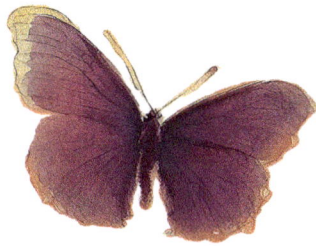

A NOTE FROM
THE PUBLISHER

When I first began publishing books in December 2008, I prayed a very intentional prayer:

"Lord, send me the authors You want me to publish."

I knew from the beginning that this work was not just business, it was ministry. I believed that every story He sent my way would have purpose, and every author would be part of the assignment He was trusting me to fulfill. And over the years, I have seen that prayer answered again and again.

I also learned something important: whenever I tried to move ahead of God, choosing projects on my own or stepping outside His timing, things never seemed to flow smoothly. The process felt strained, heavy, or out of alignment. But every time I waited for the authors He chose, everything came together with clarity, ease, and peace.

Those experiences taught me to stay sensitive to God's leading, because He knows exactly whose stories He wants me to help bring into the world.

When I received the call from Yvonne, I had no idea how deeply her story would touch me. The moment she began sharing her experience, something in my spirit immediately recognized that this connection was divine. I knew God had sent her. What I didn't realize at the time was how powerfully her journey would unfold on the pages of this book.

It was the first time I had ever published a book about organ transplantation. It was new territory for me, and I wanted to approach it with accuracy, sensitivity, and complete understanding. I began researching liver transplants and quickly discovered the harsh realities African Americans have historically faced; the barriers, inequities, delays, and systemic obstacles that have too often determined who receives life-saving care and who does not. Learning this made Yvonne's survival even more extraordinary. Her journey was not just a medical victory; it was a victory over history itself.

I put together an outline and sent it to Yvonne, hoping it would help guide the writing. Not only did she embrace it, but she immediately poured her heart, her testimony, and her truth into every question I asked. Her willingness, her openness, and her spirit of cooperation made the process a blessing.

It was during one of our initial conversations that she told me **Pastor Joyce Jay of Worship Life Center in Mesa, Arizona,** had referred her to me. Years earlier, I had published Pastor Joyce Jay's book, *The Power of OK*. Hearing that Yvonne was sent to me through someone whose ministry and message I already respected was yet another confirmation that God was orchestrating this connection long before I ever picked up the phone.

As I continued reading Yvonne's responses, I felt something else, a deep admiration for her strength and her character. Despite everything she had endured, she had the sweetest spirit, the kindest disposition, and a level of grace that only someone who walks closely with God could possess. The more I read, the more I realized she was an Evangelist herself. And suddenly, everything made sense.

Her peace.

Her faith.

Her endurance.

Her ability to remain gentle even when life had been anything but gentle to her.

Yvonne wasn't just telling a story; she was living a testimony.

Publishing this book has reminded me once again that God still writes miracles into everyday lives. He still aligns paths. He still sends people with stories that carry healing and purpose. And sometimes, He allows us to be part of bringing those stories into the world.

As you read this book, I pray you will feel what I felt, awe at God's goodness, admiration for Yvonne's courage, and a renewed belief that miracles still happen. Her journey is living proof that even in the darkest valleys, God is there. He sees us. He sustains us. And He will carry us through.

—*Willa Robinson*
Publisher, KP Publishing Company

"I shall not die, but live, and declare the works of the Lord."
—Psalm 118:17 (KJV)

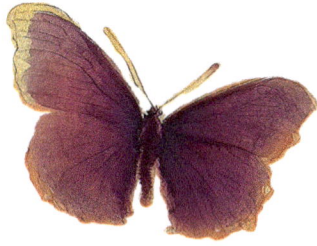

FOREWORD

It is a profound honor to write this foreword, not only as Yvonne Weaver's son, but as one who has witnessed the extraordinary resilience of her spirit and the enduring power of her faith. For more than twenty three years, I walked alongside my mother through the reality of chronic liver disease, serving as her caregiver, her advocate, and often her strongest source of encouragement. Even after the lifesaving gift of a liver transplant, I stood with her through the emotional and spiritual challenges of healing, including the depression that can accompany long term recovery. Through every season, her strength became my lesson, and her faith became my foundation.

In 2015, I published *Transforming the Minds of Men: Maximizing Potential from Childhood to Manhood,* a work focused on understanding how transformation occurs when principles are applied to real life. While that book centers on men, it is important to acknowledge that the strength I wrote about was first modeled for me by my mother. Long before I taught others about resilience, discipline, and purpose, I watched those qualities lived out daily in her life. She sowed seeds of faith, perseverance, and courage that now allow me to inspire, teach, and lead others with authenticity and conviction.

As a pastor for more than twenty one years, first serving in Mesa, Arizona with Impacted for Purpose Ministries and now for the past decade at Greater New Hope Baptist Church in High Point, North Carolina, I have come to understand that transformation is rarely instantaneous. It is formed through sustained faithfulness, tested endurance, and a willingness to trust God even when outcomes are uncertain. Yvonne's story embodies this truth. Her journey demonstrates that faith is not passive belief, but active trust practiced day by day.

This book is not simply a medical memoir. It is a living testimony of applied faith. It reveals how belief, when exercised under pressure, becomes a source of healing and hope. Yvonne does not present a polished narrative of victory without struggle. Instead, she offers an honest account of endurance, reminding readers that God's work often unfolds gradually and purposefully.

Her life reflects the rhythms of the Christian walk. There are seasons of waiting, moments of fear, and periods of renewal. Yet through it all, her faith remained anchored in God's promises. She trusted not only for healing of the body, but for restoration of the mind and spirit as well.

To the reader, I offer this encouragement. Approach these pages with openness and expectancy. Allow this story to speak into your own journey. May it strengthen your faith, deepen your perseverance, and remind you that transformation is possible when faith is lived, not merely confessed. This book stands as evidence that a life rooted in faith can sow seeds that bless generations.

Lovelle McMichael
Pastor, Greater New Hope Baptist Church

Author, *Transforming the Minds of Men:*
Maximizing Potential from Childhood to Manhood

*"I shall not die, but live,
and declare the works of the Lord."*
Psalm 118:17 (NKJV)

A Living Testimony

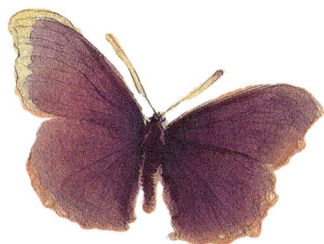

INTRODUCTION

In May 1995, I developed a red, inflamed rash across my cheeks and the bridge of my nose—what doctors call a "butterfly rash" because of its shape. It felt hot, slightly painful, and rough to the touch. I didn't know it then, but this rash is often associated with Systemic Lupus Erythematosus (SLE). After additional testing, I was officially diagnosed with lupus that same year.

Not long after, I noticed unusual bleeding beneath my fingernail beds. My doctor ordered blood work to determine whether I could tolerate a prescribed medication—but when the results came back, the concern shifted. I was told I couldn't take the medication because my liver numbers were elevated. I was referred to a hepatologist, and after further tests, I was diagnosed with a rare liver disease called Primary Sclerosing Cholangitis (PSC).

Two life-altering autoimmune diseases in less than a year—lupus and PSC. That's when I began to wonder: had I been misdiagnosed at first?

Or did I truly have both? The symptoms of lupus and PSC can overlap—fatigue, joint pain, abnormal bloodwork—and PSC is so rare that it's often discovered after something else is suspected. To this day, I'm still not sure whether one masked the other or whether they always coexisted inside me.

At that time, I was told I wasn't eligible for the liver transplant list because my M.E.L.D. score (Model for End-Stage Liver Disease) wasn't high enough. The M.E.L.D. score ranges from 6 (less ill) to 40 (gravely ill); mine was only 9. But my doctors warned me that PSC would inevitably progress, and I would eventually need a liver transplant.

In September 2004, I moved from Philadelphia to Mesa, Arizona, seeking a fresh start and access to better care. My younger son and his wife lived in Mesa, so I would not be alone. I was blessed with a job almost immediately when I arrived in Arizona through a longtime friend from Philadelphia who had been there for years. I resumed my care at Mayo Clinic Hospital, where they continue the evaluations for a possible Liver transplant. I remained under their care until February 2009, when I lost my job because I was at the top of the layoff list, and along with it, my medical insurance. Looking back, I see this journey not just as a series of medical diagnoses—but as a testimony of survival, faith, and perseverance in the face of uncertainty. Even though I still suffered from fatigue and pain regularly, I still looked for work and was able to secure another job as a data entry clerk at an insurance company.

I have always been a hard worker because I had three growing sons whom I cared for as a single mom, and I wanted them to see an example of no excuses, so I had to survive no matter what.

I was a hairstylist for over 30 years at our family salon, and I also worked at group homes for boys ages 13 to 18 on the weekends after my sons became adults and moved out. In 1998, I began a Daycare for children ages, infant to five years old, until I moved to Arizona. My spiritual mother taught us to see the good in every situation.

"For the joy of the LORD is your strength."
Nehemiah 8:10 (KJV)

*"For I will restore health to you
And heal you of your wounds,"*
says the Lord.
Jeremiah 30:17 (NKJV)

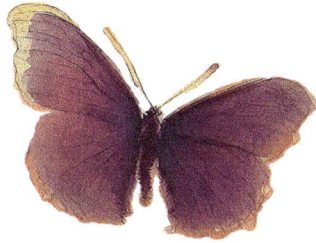

CHAPTER ONE

TRUSTING THE PROCESS

I had no insurance and couldn't get state assistance because, at the time, I was making too much with unemployment (go figure). As my health deteriorated, I sought help at a free clinic in Mesa that operated out of a church. When I arrived, the line was long. After a while, a clinic worker stepped outside, began counting patients, and cut off the line right at me.

I pleaded with them to let me in, but they couldn't take any more patients that day. Defeated, I returned home and did what I always did. I talked to the Lord. Once again, He told me, *"Trust Me."*

The pain was unbearable. Every night, I placed a heating pad on my stomach, it was the only way I could get any sleep.

One day, my son had had enough. "Mom, I'm taking you to the emergency room. You've been in pain long enough. We'll deal with insurance later."

He took me to Banner Baywood Hospital in Mesa, where they admitted me. The doctors ran multiple tests but found nothing conclusive. Because I had no insurance, the hospital staff wanted to discharge me.

The next day, a doctor came to check on me. She sat on the edge of my bed and gently said, *"I see you don't have insurance."* I explained my struggles with trying to get state assistance. She looked at me with determination and said, *"If I have to keep you here until your hospital expenses outweigh your income, I will."*

And she did just that.

God always has a ram in the bush. Thanks to the hospital's social worker, I was able to get insurance through state assistance. With coverage finally in place, I started seeking new doctors and specialists.

I began seeing doctors within the Banner Healthcare System. Across the board, they were excellent—from my primary care doctor to the numerous specialists who were attentive and worked closely together regarding my health.

In April 2008, my fatigue worsened. I had no energy, and the pain became unbearable. Once again, my son took me to the ER.

The ER doctor determined that I needed emergency gallbladder removal surgery. My son and I prayed. Then, by what I can only describe as divine intervention, my gastroenterologist, whom I had an appointment with the following week, was on call in the ER that night. He came to examine me, looked at the test that was already taken, and delivered a life-saving decision.

"There will be no emergency surgery," he said. *"Your system is septic."*

What a mighty God we serve! Had I consented to the emergency surgery, I could have died from the infection in my body.

After days of monitoring and treatment, once the infection was under control, doctors successfully removed my gallbladder. For the first time in a long while, I started feeling better. My MELD score remained low, and my strength began to return.

My primary physician, Dr. Chuba Ononye (Internal Medicine), had referred me to Dr. David Tessler (Gastroenterologist), the same doctor who prevented my emergency surgery. These two worked together diligently, eventually introducing me to Dr. Richard Manch (now retired) at Banner Good Samaritan, which is now Banner University in Phoenix, Arizona.

It wasn't until August 2018 that I met Dr. Nathan Rohit and my transplant team. By then, my MELD score had risen enough for me to be placed on the transplant list.

It's astonishing how, when you don't have the best insurance, or if the state or hospital system you're in doesn't allow living donors, you practically have to be at death's door to receive a chance at survival.

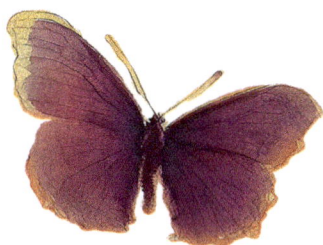

CHAPTER TWO

EMOTIONAL ROLLERCOASTER

DEALING WITH FEAR AND ANXIETY

"For God has not given us a spirit of fear, but of power, and of love, and of a sound mind."

2 Timothy 1:7

Looking back, I can honestly say that I was never consumed by fear or anxiety because of my condition. I was blessed to have two praying grandmothers who lived by faith, not just in words but in action. They taught me to trust in God, leaning on His promises (Proverbs 3:5-6).

If I'm being truthful, when I first heard my diagnosis, fear and nervousness crept in. That initial reaction was only natural. But I refused to let fear take root. I would remind myself of my grandmothers' unwavering faith and the lessons they instilled in me. As I prayed, *the peace of God, which surpasses all understanding, would wash over me* (Philippians 4:7).

Accepting my diagnosis was a journey. I had to face the reality that my condition was irreversible without a transplant. There were only two options:

1. A living donor transplant, where a portion of a healthy person's liver would replace the damaged part of mine.

2. A full transplant, which meant waiting until my liver failed completely and hoping for a compatible donor.

The uncertainty was overwhelming at times, but I refused to live in fear. Instead, I chose to trust God for the outcome and continue living my life to the fullest.

I am beyond blessed with a strong support system. My three sons had seen me care for my grandparents (their great-grandparents), and they had helped me care for them as well. That same love and devotion were now extended to me.

My father (now deceased), his siblings, my sons and daughter-in-loves, my grandchildren, and my sisters in Christ all stood by me. My daughter-in-love, Angie, played a vital role in organizing family support. She made sure that my husband, Dennis, and I were never alone during this journey. From the moment I was admitted to the hospital to my recovery at home, there was always someone by my side.

At the time, I did not have the opportunity to connect with other transplant survivors. However, I knew that God had surrounded me with the support I needed.

Because my memory had significantly declined due to my illness, my son Lovelle and Angie walked through the transplant process with me. They attended appointments, asked questions, and made sure I understood what was happening.

From them, I learned that I had an important role to play. I had to do my part by staying as healthy as possible. This meant being mindful of my diet and staying active, even when I didn't feel up to it.

Lifestyle changes weren't a choice, they were a necessity. Long before my transplant, I had already slowed down. Fatigue often kept me from doing the things I once loved.

However, I refused to let my condition completely dictate my life. I remained as active as my body allowed. When I felt exhausted, I rested. But when I had the strength, I moved. My body may have been failing, but my spirit remained strong.

"Lord my God,
I called to you for help,
and you healed me."
Psalm 30:2 (NIV)

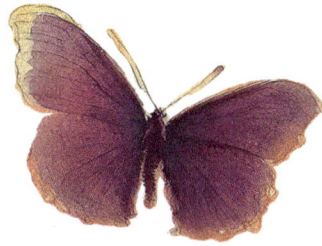

CHAPTER THREE

THE TRANSPLANT PROCESS

Waiting for a transplant is unlike anything else. It's a journey filled with faith, uncertainty, and surrender. It's a season of trusting God for the unknown while preparing for the possibility of life-changing surgery. My journey to receiving a liver was filled with highs and lows, but through it all, God's hand was evident.

In August 2018, I was admitted to the hospital, and it was only then that I was officially placed on the transplant waiting list. My doctors told me that I would have to stay in the hospital until a liver became available. There was no going home, no waiting in the comfort of my own bed, just an indefinite period of hospital stays, medical evaluations, and waiting.

The waiting process brought natural waves of anxiety. Thoughts of life and death were inevitable— *Would I live long enough to receive a liver?* But I refused to let fear take hold of me. Instead, I held tightly to the words God had spoken to me at the beginning of this journey:

"What you are going through is not for you, but so that others will see Me through you."

I knew that whatever happened, my testimony would glorify God.

On September 6th, my son, Pastor Lovelle McMichael Sr., started a a prayer line. Family, friends, and believers from all over the world joined in—reading scriptures, offering words of encouragement, and lifting me up in prayer.

Then, in the early morning hours of September 7th, at 3:45 a.m. my phone rang.

Before I could even process what was happening, my daughter-in-love, Angie, turned to me and said, *"That better be someone calling about a liver at this time of the morning."*

Hallelujah—it was!

The voice on the other end said, *"We have a potential donor. Of course, we need to confirm that the liver is in good condition."* The donor was classified as a standard criteria donor—brain dead, with no high-risk factors. After thorough testing, the liver was deemed viable for transplant. Immediately, my medical team began running tests to prepare me for surgery.

By 10:30 a.m. on September 10, 2018, I was prepped. As I was wheeled to the operating room, my husband, my spiritual sister, Shirley Lewis, my eldest son Eric, and Angie were by my side. We prayed together before they rolled me into surgery.

Won't He do it!

The procedure lasted five hours. Though I was unconscious, I later learned how precise and intricate the transplant process was. Every step was critical. Every decision a matter of life or death.

When I woke up after surgery, I was in the ICU. The doctors and nurses had intentionally kept me sedated to allow my body to rest and prevent clotting. I was connected to multiple medical devices, including an arterial line, a central line for fluids and medications, a heart catheter, and a breathing tube.

Even in my groggy state, I felt an overwhelming sense of gratitude, not only for my life but for the incredible team of surgeons, nurses, and staff at Banner University Hospital who cared for me with such dedication.

Most importantly, I was, and still am, deeply grateful for my donor and their family. Their loss gave me life. Though I reached out to express my thanks, I have not received a response. Still, I pray for them continually, knowing that their sacrifice changed my life forever.

Yet, I also recognize that not every healing story ends this way.

For me, healing came in the form of another chance at life. But for others, healing comes in going home to be with the Lord.

> *"We are confident, I say, and willing rather to be absent from the body, and to be present with the Lord."*
>
> 2 Corinthians 5:8

> *"For to me, to live is Christ, and to die is gain."*
>
> Philippians 1:21

The days following my transplant were some of the hardest of my life. I remained in the hospital until October, requiring multiple blood transfusions and learning how to walk again. My body had become so weak that standing unassisted was impossible.

I hadn't realized just how close to death I had been. This experience made me appreciate the simple things we often take for granted—like the ability to get out of bed, walk to the restroom, or take a shower without assistance.

At first, walking from my hospital bed to the hallway drained every bit of energy I had. But with determination, I made progress, first walking one lap around the nurses' station, then three laps, and eventually, the entire hospital floor.

By November, I could care for myself again. *What a blessing!*

As a post-transplant patient, my new reality included a strict medication regimen.

For the first three years, I took 2mg of Prograf (Tacrolimus) twice daily at 8 a.m. and 8 p.m. In the fourth year, my dosage was reduced to 1mg twice a day, then to 0.5mg in the morning and 1mg at night. This is my seventh year, and I now take 1 mg twice a day. I received a good report from the doctor recently, and now I am getting blood work done every three months as opposed to once a month.

Thankfully, I have not experienced significant side effects, though my doctors made adjustments when necessary. But through it all, I have learned to pray over my medicine before I take it:

"Father, I thank You for this medication. Let it serve its purpose and no more. Remove anything harmful, and bless the hands that prepared it. In Jesus' name, Amen."

This journey has changed me forever. It has deepened my faith, strengthened my resolve, and given me a new perspective on life.

One of the most powerful lessons I've learned is that faith is not just about believing, it's about trusting God daily, no matter the outcome.

There were many things I had to learn throughout this experience:

- To *"hold my peace and let the Lord fight my battles."*

  Exodus 14:14

- To *"be still and know that He is God."*

  Psalm 46:10

- To *"be swift to hear, slow to speak, and slow to wrath."*

  James 1:19

- To *"put on the full armor of God every day before stepping into the world."*

  Ephesians 6:10-18 (NIV)

- And most importantly, to *pause, think, and pray before reacting*—a lesson from my spiritual mother that I still practice to this day.

Another lesson?

"Treat people the way you want to be treated."

This requires intentional effort every single day. And I made a life-changing decision:

"I have a good day every day—by choice."

I haven't always felt this way. I've had my share of bad days—enough of them to realize that choosing joy is always worth it.

"Choose for yourselves this day whom you will serve..."
Joshua 24:15 (NKJV)

I have lived through suffering. I have witnessed God's miracles firsthand. And now, I am grateful for every moment.

"He comforts us in all our troubles so that we can comfort others."
2 Corinthians 1:4 (NLT)

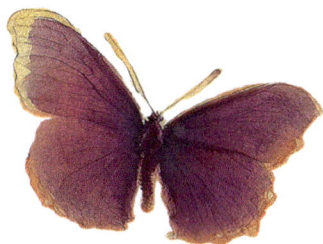

CHAPTER FOUR

OVERCOMING OBSTACLES

Healing doesn't happen overnight. It takes time. It happens from the inside out, both physically and spiritually. In the months after my transplant, I was grateful for every step forward, even the small ones. Every day that I woke up, I gave God the glory because I knew that every breath, every moment of strength, was a gift. Tomorrow is not promised to any of us, and I didn't want to waste any opportunity to spend time with my family.

My husband and I traveled to California to visit my son, Shariff, and his family for Thanksgiving. It was a beautiful time, filled with love, laughter, and the warmth of family. Our extended relatives who lived in California came to celebrate, making it a truly special holiday.

Then, in December, I traveled to North Carolina to visit my son Lovelle and his family. Meanwhile, my husband went to Detroit to spend Christmas with his loved ones. Though we were apart, our hearts were full. I even celebrated my birthday while I was there, grateful for another year of life.

As instructed by my doctor, I went to get my routine bloodwork done after the holidays. That's when things took an unexpected turn. My results were concerning, and I was immediately taken to Duke University Medical Center in Raleigh, North Carolina. What was supposed to be a short visit turned into a hospital stay from December 2019 until the end of February 2020.

When I was admitted to Duke University, the transplant team explained to me that they typically do not take on transplant cases that are under a year old. But then, *God stepped in.*

God gave me favor, and they took on my case.

Hallelujah!

Because of my condition, I was required to remain in North Carolina for an entire year before it was safe for me to travel again. That year was from February 2019 until March 2020.

By March 2020, just as the COVID-19 pandemic was beginning to shut down the world, I knew I needed to get home. I had been away from my husband for over a year. Though he visited me as often as possible, the time apart had been difficult.

With the help of my children, I was able to secure a plane ticket. I returned home to my husband just before travel restrictions were enforced due to the pandemic.

September 10, 2025, I celebrated my seven-year "LiverVersary."

God is so amazing!

When I look back over all that I have been through—from the day I was diagnosed until now—there is only one thing I can say: *"Won't He Do It?!"*

Through these last 28 years, I have learned some valuable lessons, and I am still learning. My grandmother always reminded me that God is constantly shaping our character, and that process lasts a lifetime.

I am eternally grateful for every lesson, every trial, and every moment of grace. My hope is that these pages of my journey will inspire and encourage you to believe that no matter what you go through in life:

"I can do all things through Christ who strengthens me."
Philippians 4:13 (NKJV)

There is so much I do not remember from before August 2018, especially in the weeks following my surgery. But I am grateful for my family, who kept detailed notes and updates.

My daughter-in-love, Angie, started a journal on CaringBridge.com, recording every step of my journey. She sent out updates to the family, ensuring that everyone stayed informed about my condition.

One of the messages sent to my family on **July 17, 2018**, read:

"Mother Dear was taken to the hospital last night with a temp of 102. She just got put in a room. Lower bowel obstruction inflammation with possible infection. Catheter and tube going through her nose into her belly (very uncomfortable). Temp is down to 98. Prayers up."

Though I don't remember much from that time, these notes remind me of just how much I went through, and how God carried me through every moment.

Angie's updates helped document my progress:

- Fluid retention was improving—800ML had been drained the previous week, showing progress.

- Sodium levels were lowering.

- Bilirubin levels remained high, causing itching, but the doctors assured us that healing takes time.

- Sharp stomach pains persisted, likely due to bowel and bladder issues.

- I was prescribed magnesium to help with cramping in my legs and feet.

One of the biggest concerns at the time was my MELD score—the score that determines how sick a liver transplant patient is. At that time, my MELD score was 20 (patients with scores of 40+ are considered critical).

The doctors suggested that I be re-evaluated for transplant eligibility. However, because living donor transplants hadn't been done in Arizona for five years, the options were extremely limited.

Travel was still possible, but my doctors advised that I should never travel alone. Liver transplant patients can become confused or disoriented, and I needed someone with me who understood my condition and could recognize the signs if something were wrong.

As my transplant evaluation process continued, the team coordinated with insurance, financial departments, and transplant specialists to determine my next steps. My family rallied around me, making sure someone was always available to help.

#GodStillWorksMiracles

Through all of these challenges, one scripture remained close to my heart:

"I shall not die, but live, and declare the works of the LORD."
Psalm 118:17

Even in my weakest moments, I refused to give up. One of the greatest lessons I learned during this time was **to be still and trust God.**

"Be still and know that I am God."
Psalm 46:10

After my transplant, I was feeling good, so I moved too fast. I should have listened to my body and waited before traveling. But even in my missteps, God's mercy and grace kept me. I am forever grateful to Duke University Medical Center for taking on my case when others wouldn't.

This journey has taught me more than I could have ever imagined. It has strengthened my faith, deepened my understanding of patience, and reminded me of the power of resilience.

Though healing is a process, I know that every challenge I faced was a part of my testimony.

There were times when I questioned why I had to go through so much. But now, looking back, I see how every trial was shaping me —preparing me to share this testimony and encouraging others to trust in God's plan.

I know that if you're reading this, you may be facing your own struggles. You may feel like your healing is taking too long, or that your obstacles are too great.

But let me tell you this: God is not finished with you yet.

"I can do all things through Christ who strengthens me."
Philippians 4:13

No matter what you are going through, trust that God is writing your story, just as He has written mine.

*"My flesh and my heart may fail,
but God is the strength of my heart
and my portion forever."*
Psalm 73:26 (NIV)

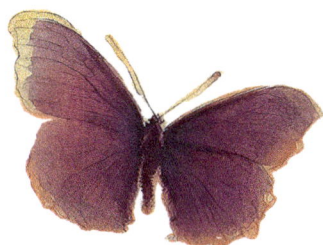

CHAPTER FIVE

THE SUPPORT SYSTEM

No one walks through life alone. Whether in moments of joy or seasons of struggle, we all need people who stand by us, uplift us, and help carry the burdens we cannot bear alone.

When I think about the phenomenal support system God has blessed me with, I am overwhelmed with gratitude. My heart swells with emotion as I reflect on the unwavering love, prayers, and sacrifices that carried me through this journey.

I did not walk this road alone. God surrounded me with family, friends, compassionate medical professionals, and a loving community who stood with me every step of the way.

From the very beginning, my family and friends became my lifeline. Their prayers covered me. Their presence strengthened me. Their unwavering faith carried me through my darkest days.

My three sons, Eric, Shariff, and Lovelle, stood by me in ways I can never fully express myself. They had already witnessed me care for their great-grandparents, and now, without hesitation, they cared for me in the same way.

Each of them, along with my extended family, took turns traveling from Philadelphia, North Carolina, California, and locally in Arizona to be with me. They never left my side, and no matter how far away they were, they always found a way to show up—physically, emotionally, and spiritually.

The sacrifices my family made for me cannot be measured. They took time off work, spent weeks at a time helping me recover, and even covered expenses to make sure I had everything I needed.

My daughter-in-love, Angie, played a particularly instrumental role in keeping everyone informed, ensuring I was never alone, and taking care of countless details that I couldn't manage on my own. She updated my family, kept track of my medical information, and helped coordinate support from across the country.

My husband, Dennis, was my rock. Even in the times we had to be apart due to my medical care, he remained steadfast and supportive, doing everything he could to make sure I was taken care of.

There was never a moment when we felt abandoned. We were always surrounded by love, support, and encouragement. I can never thank my family enough. No words will ever be enough to express my gratitude.

Beyond my family, I was also blessed with an exceptional team of healthcare providers who played a crucial role in my survival and recovery. The doctors, nurses, and specialists at Banner University in Arizona and Duke University in North Carolina were not only skilled professionals, they were compassionate caregivers who treated me with kindness, dignity, and respect.

When you're fighting for your life, trust in your medical team is everything. I had two phenomenal transplant teams, one in Arizona and one in North Carolina, and both went above and beyond to ensure I received the best possible care.

They didn't just see me as a patient, they saw me as a person, a woman with a family, faith, and a future worth fighting for. From answering my questions with patience to making sure I was comfortable during painful procedures, their dedication reassured me that I was in the best hands possible. I am forever grateful for their expertise, their kindness, and their commitment to my healing.

Support doesn't only come from family and medical professionals, it also comes from the people around you. The community where I live in Arizona has been incredibly supportive throughout my journey. Even today, they continue to check in on me, encourage me, and remind me that I am never alone.

One of the greatest blessings of this journey has been the opportunity to connect with other transplant recipients. Speaking with people who understand the struggles, fears, and victories that come with transplantation is a powerful source of strength and encouragement.

There is something deeply comforting about being able to talk to someone who has walked the same road, who knows what it feels like to wait for a transplant, to undergo surgery, and to live with the daily reality of anti-rejection medication and follow-up care. These connections remind me that I am part of a larger story—a community of survivors who share in the miracle of another chance at life.

This experience has also ignited in me a passion for organ donation advocacy. If there is one thing my journey has reinforced, it is the critical need for organ donors.

One selfless decision can save multiple lives.

My donor's gift gave me another chance. Their family's sacrifice changed my life forever. I now advocate for organ donation awareness, encouraging others to register as donors so that more lives can be saved.

Every person who chooses to give the gift of life becomes a part of a story greater than their own.

Through it all, my faith in God was the anchor that held me steady. I leaned on Him in my weakest moments, and He surrounded me with the right people at the right time to walk this journey with me.

The prayers of my family, friends, and even strangers were a constant source of strength. I am a witness that God hears the cries of His people.

Even when I didn't know what the future held, I knew who held my future.

Looking back, I see that I was never alone. God surrounded me with family, friends, medical professionals, and a loving community to help me through this journey. Their support was a testament to the power of love, faith, and human kindness.

I am alive today because of the sacrifices, prayers, and dedication of so many people. And I will spend the rest of my life paying that love forward—in my words, my actions, and my testimony.

> *"Bear one another's burdens, and so fulfill the law of Christ."*
> Galatians 6:2 (ESV)

I pray that if you are going through a difficult season, you find strength in those around you. You are not alone. There are people who love you, people who will walk this journey with you, and a God who will never leave your side.

And if you ever doubt the power of community, just remember my story, because I am a walking, talking miracle.

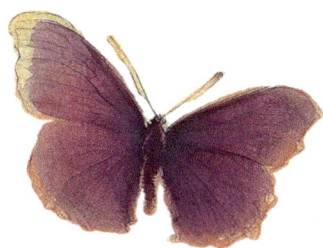

LIVING THE MIRACLE

The following images capture the journey of life renewed—family moments, triumphs after transplant, and blessings experienced along the way. Each photo is a reminder that every day is truly a gift.

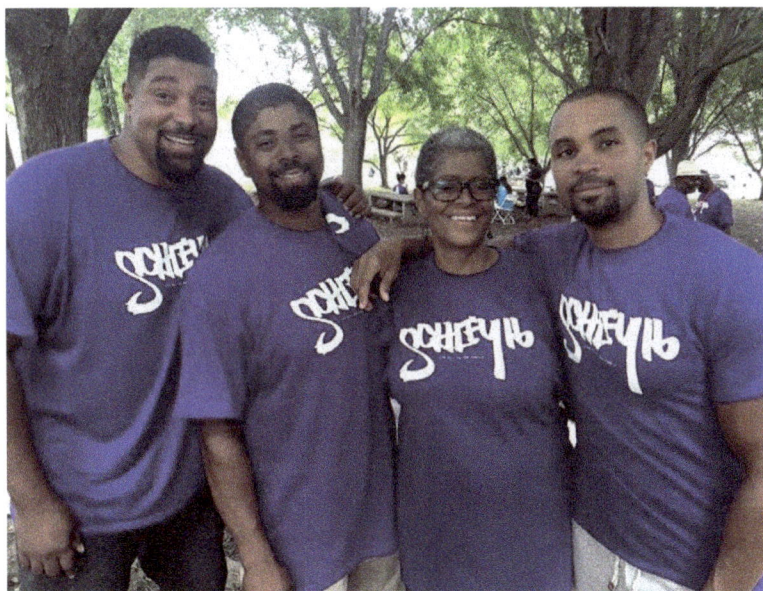

Family Reunion 2016

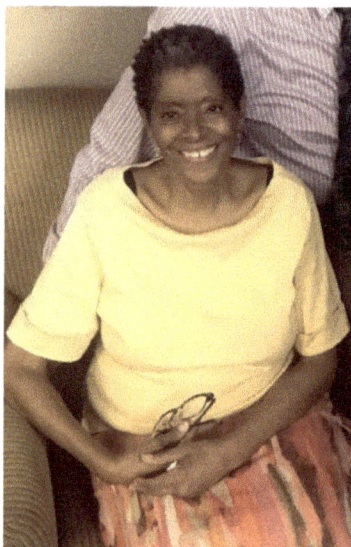

Evangelist Yvonne
May 2018

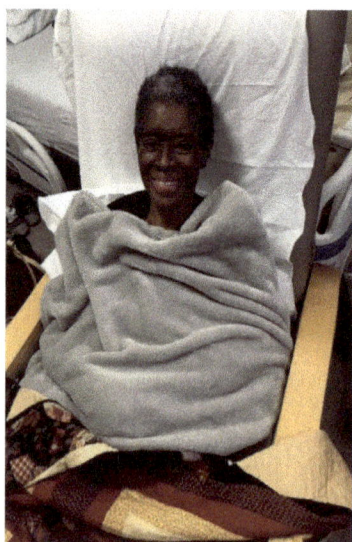

Yvonne
Before the transplant 2018

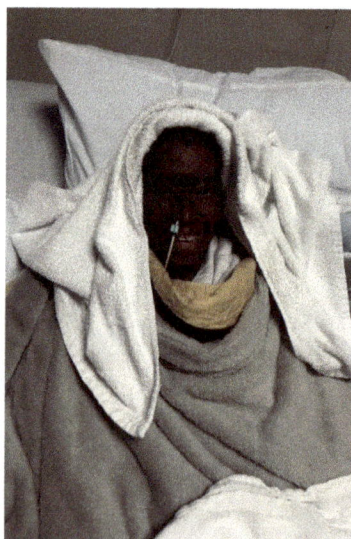

Yvonne
After the transplant 2018

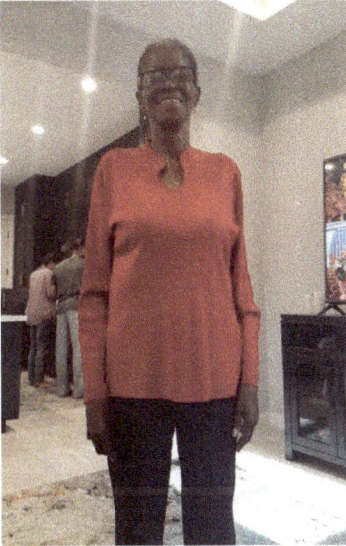

Yvonne
December 2018

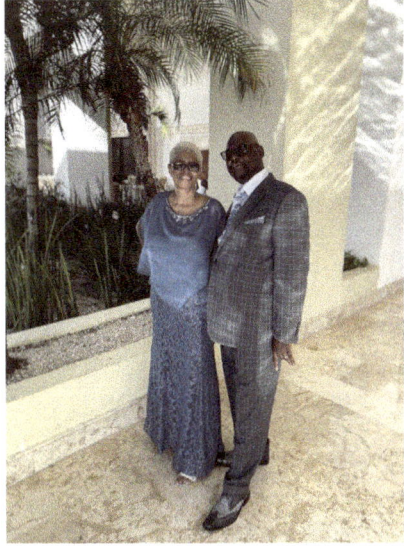

Yvonne and husband, Dennis,
Cancun 2020

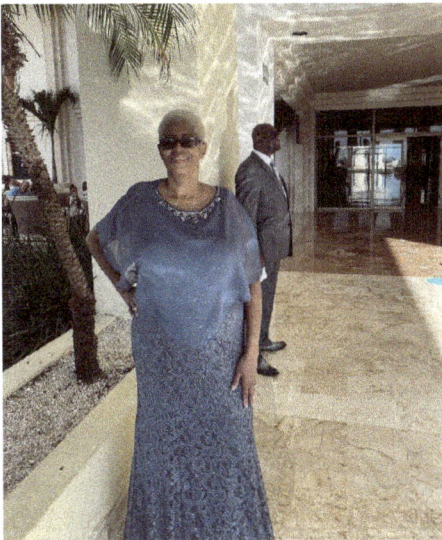

Yvonne - Cancun, November 2020
Husband, Dennis, in the background.

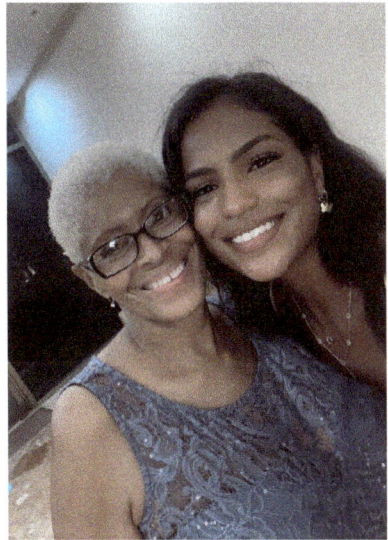

Yvonne, and granddaughter, Monet,
Cancun November 2020

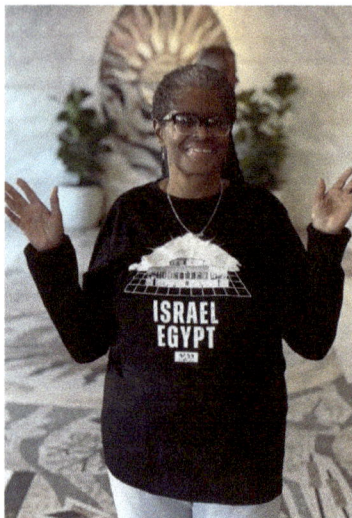

Yvonne
Israel December 2022

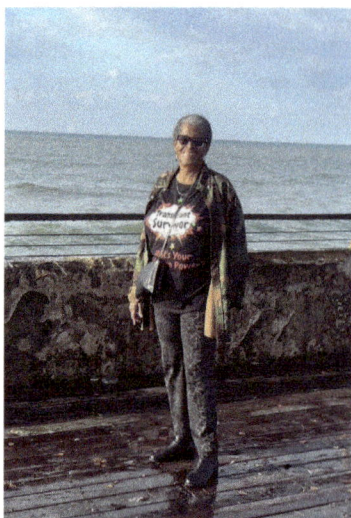

Yvonne
Egypt December 2022

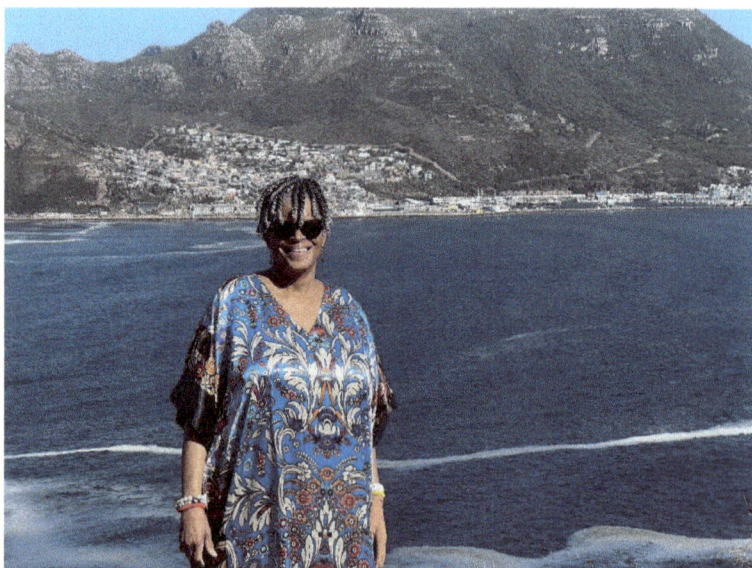

Yvonne
South Africa December 2024

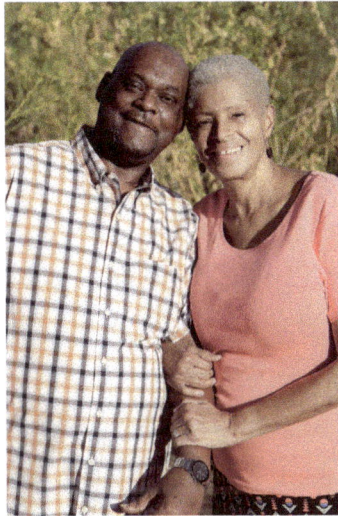

Yvonne
and husband, Dennis

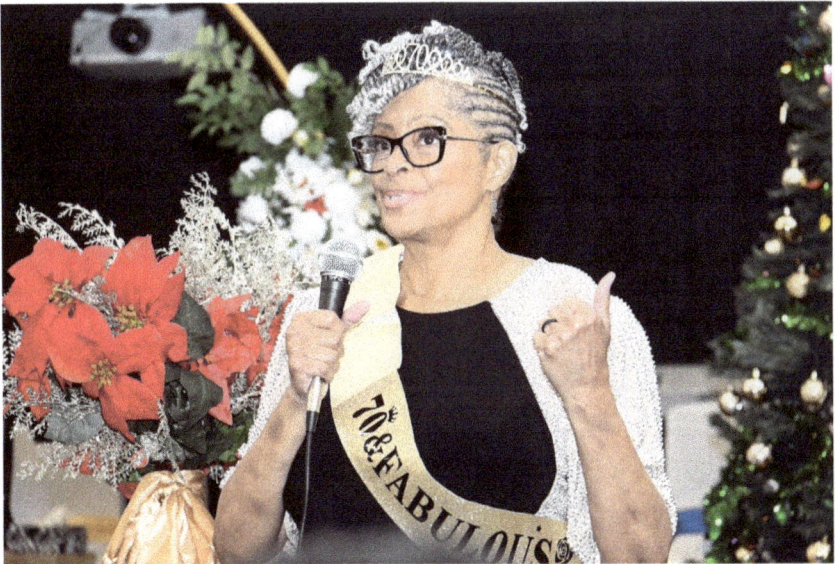

Yvonne
70th Birthday Celebration

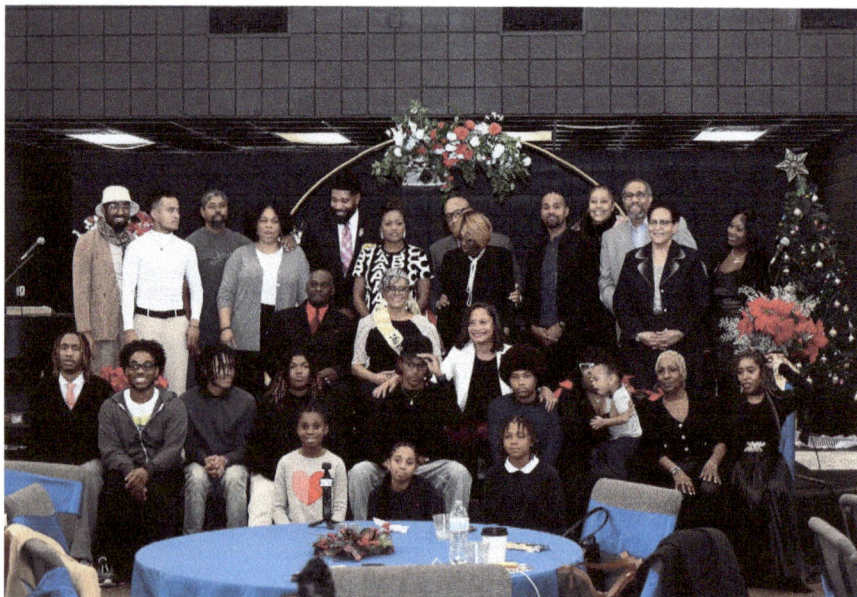

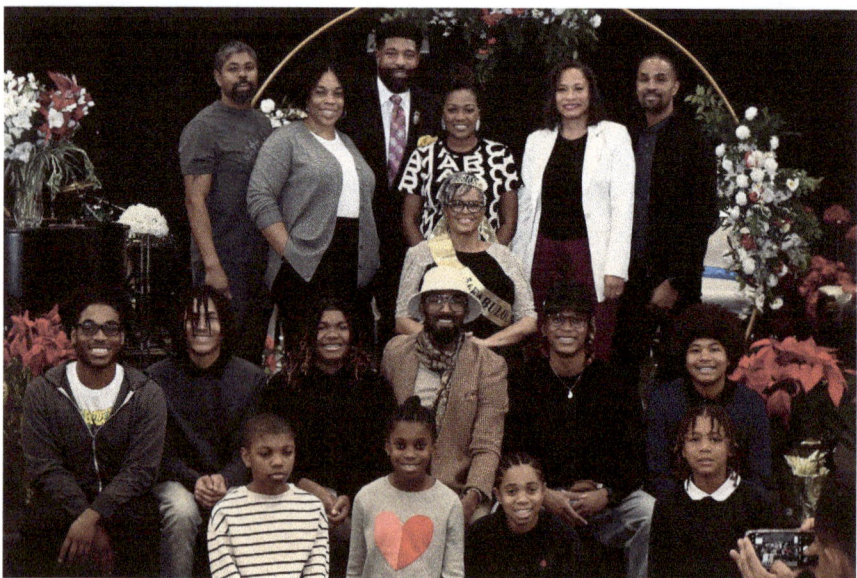

Yvonne
70th Birthday Celebration

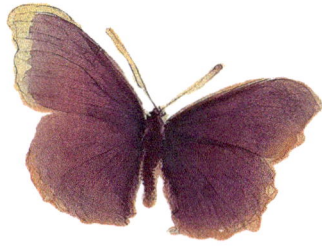

CHAPTER SIX

A NEW LEASE ON LIFE

There is no greater gift than the gift of life itself. Each day I wake up, I do so with a grateful heart, knowing that I have been given another chance—another opportunity to live, love, and fulfill the purpose God has placed within me.

Surviving a life-threatening illness changes everything. It shifts your perspective, sharpens your priorities, and deepens your appreciation for the small, beautiful moments that many take for granted. I have learned not to waste time, not to put off what is important, and to cherish every experience, whether big or small.

"Whereas ye know not what shall be on the morrow. For what is your life? It is even a vapor, that appeareth for a little time, and then vanisheth away."

James 4:14

I give thanks to God every single day for allowing me to live. My heart overflows with gratitude, not just for another chance but for the strength, wisdom, and renewed sense of purpose that have come through my journey.

I no longer take anything for granted. The ability to wake up, to breathe without pain, to walk without struggle, and to simply exist in the presence of my loved ones. These are gifts, not entitlements.

One of the greatest blessings of my life is my family—my many grandchildren. From the ages of 30 to three years old, they are the light of my life. Every time I see their faces, I am reminded that I fought to live not just for myself, but for them too.

I want to be here to watch them grow up, to celebrate their victories, to wipe their tears, and to be the source of wisdom and love that they can always turn to.

Life is precious, and I am determined to embrace every single moment with joy, purpose, and an open heart.

Another chance at life means a second chance to dream, to plan, and to pursue the things that truly matter.

When I was fighting for my life, my only goal was survival. But now that I have been given this miraculous gift, I refuse to simply exist, I want to thrive.

I have set new goals and aspirations, pushing myself to step into the fullness of the life God has granted me. I wake up each morning with the desire to give back, to help others, and to use my testimony to inspire and encourage those who are facing their own struggles.

What is the point of being given another chance if I don't use it to make a difference?

I now dedicate myself to:

- Encouraging transplant patients—helping them navigate the emotional and physical challenges that come with the journey.

- Advocating for organ donation—sharing my story so that more people will understand the importance of registering as donors.

- Spreading the message of faith and resilience—reminding others that no matter how dark the storm, God is still in control.

This is my new lease on life, and I am determined to make the most of every moment. Not everyone gets another chance. Not everyone who fought the battle that I fought made it through. I do not take this gift lightly, and I will spend the rest of my life honoring it.

I pray that my story serves as a reminder to cherish each day, to love fully, to dream boldly, and to walk in gratitude.

God has kept me here for a reason, and I will spend every breath I have living out that purpose.

> *"This is the day which the Lord hath made; we will rejoice and be glad in it."*
>
> Psalm 118:24

And rejoice, I will.

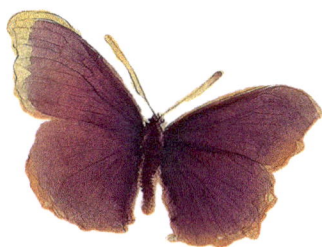

CHAPTER SEVEN

THE OUTCOME

As I look back over the last 28 years, I can see just how much I have been through. The challenges, the battles, the setbacks, and the victories have all shaped me into the person I am today.

This journey has not been easy, but through it all, I have learned some valuable lessons. One of the most important lessons is learning to manage my mindset.

So much of what we face—our struggles, our healing, our victories—begins in the mind. If we allow doubt, fear, and negativity to take hold, they will cripple us before the battle even begins. But when we choose faith over fear, we begin to see God's hand moving in ways we never imagined.

> "Don't worry about anything; instead, pray about everything; tell God your needs, and don't forget to thank him for his answers. If you do this, you will experience God's peace, which is far more wonderful than the human mind can understand. His peace will keep your thoughts and your hearts quiet and at rest as you trust in Christ Jesus."
>
> Philippians 4:6-7 (TLB)

Healing, whether physical, emotional, or spiritual, begins in the mind. A positive mindset, rooted in faith, is essential. I have learned that I must be intentional about my thoughts, focusing on what is good, what is true, and what brings peace.

> "Fix your thoughts on what is true and good and right. Think about things that are pure and lovely, and dwell on the fine, good things in others. Think about all you can praise God for and be glad about."
>
> Philippians 4:8 (TLB)

No matter how difficult life gets, I have trained myself to focus on God's goodness rather than the obstacles in front of me. That mindset has carried me through the hardest of days.

Patience is another lesson I have had to learn, both with myself and with others. Not everyone will understand your journey. Not everyone will move at the same pace. And not everyone will take the lessons from their trials the way you might. I have learned that each person's process is their own.

For me, there were lessons I had to learn the hard way. Some tests I had to take over and over again because I didn't learn the lesson the first time. I reached a point where I prayed, *"Lord, help me learn what You are trying to teach me so that I don't have to keep repeating the same test."* That prayer changed everything.

I started approaching my struggles with a different mindset. Instead of asking, *"Why is this happening to me?"* I began asking, *"What is God trying to show me through this?"*

That shift in perspective transformed the way I face challenges, and I pray it will encourage others to look for the lesson in their trials as well.

I did not go through this experience just for myself. God blessed me to live through this so that I could share His goodness with others.

When I think about the title of this book, *A Walking, Talking Miracle*—I realize just how fitting it is. Every breath I take, every step I walk, every word I speak is evidence of God's power. I shouldn't be here.

Doctors didn't expect me to make it through some of the hardest parts of this journey. There were moments when my body was failing, and the odds were stacked against me. But God had other plans.

He kept me.

He strengthened me.

And now, I have a mandate to share my story. This is my purpose—to tell the world that there is nothing too hard for God.

There is power in testimony, and I know that my story is meant to inspire, encourage, and uplift those who need to hear it.

If one person reads this and gains hope, if one person finds the strength to keep going, if one person turns to God because of what He has done in my life, then it was all worth it.

> *"With man this is impossible, but with God all things are possible."*
>
> Matthew 19:26 (NIV)

I believe that my healing and survival were not just about me. It's about helping others find hope, faith, and encouragement.

One of the ways I now do this is by advocating for organ donation. My life was saved because of the selfless act of a donor and their family.

Their gift gave me another chance, and I will always honor that by spreading awareness about the importance of organ donation.

One decision to become a donor can save multiple lives. It is an act of love, an act of generosity, and an act that can truly change someone's future.

Beyond organ donation, I also want to encourage those who are facing their own battles, whether it be an illness, a personal struggle, or an overwhelming season of uncertainty.

You are not alone.

If you are reading this and struggling with fear, doubt, or exhaustion, I want to remind you that God is still in control. No matter how impossible things seem, He has not forgotten you.

I am living proof of what happens when you keep trusting, keep believing, and keep pushing forward.

When I reflect on everything I have been through, I can only say:

"Won't He do it?!"

I am alive today not because of my own strength, but because of God's grace, mercy, and power.

If you take anything away from my story, let it be this:

God is a healer. He is a provider. He is a restorer. And He is faithful.

No matter what you are facing, hold on to your faith. Hold on to hope. And never stop believing in the miracles that only God can do.

"I shall not die, but live, and declare the works of the Lord."
Psalm 118:17

I am a walking, talking miracle—and so are you.

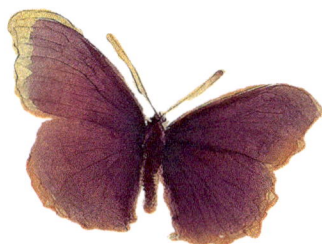

OTHER VOICES OF FAITH AND HEALING

A JOURNEY OF FAITH AND HEALING
Gloria Stinson

My need for a kidney transplant began in 1979, when I was diagnosed with an ovarian tumor. The doctors monitored it for years, but by the time I turned 57, the tumor had grown so large on the left side that it destroyed my left kidney. I lost my left kidney.

I was admitted to Bronx Lebanon Hospital for a week under a doctor's care. In the meantime, I remained under medical supervision due to a significant loss of blood. During my hospital stay, tests showed that my right kidney was functioning at only 27%. Because the tumor had damaged my left kidney and ovary, and since my husband and I were no longer planning to have children, we agreed along with my doctors, that it was best for me to have a total hysterectomy.

Emotionally and spiritually, I coped by staying busy. I became very active in my church and found joy and purpose through various roles—serving in Youth in Action, the Scholarship Program, Women United, and the Adult Choir. For years, I dedicated myself to helping others in the community, working with people in need, and surrounding myself with kind-hearted souls.

I was always tired, often asking the Lord just to give me enough strength to get through the day, and He did! With the Lord by my side, I never had to go on dialysis. Thank you, Jesus!

The most impactful part of my journey began in 2004 when my husband and I retired and moved to Arizona to be closer to family and enjoy the beautiful weather. By then, my right kidney was functioning at just 21%, which led to extreme fatigue and breathing difficulties. My body was slowing down. The doctors in Arizona advised me to get tested at the Phoenix Blood Bank and join the transplant waiting list. Beginning in 2008, I was tested twice a week—every Tuesday and Thursday. My kidney function continued to decline, nearing the danger zone of 15%.

After so many tests, I began to grow weary of the process and the travel. On Thursday, October 17, 2009, I felt like giving up hope of ever receiving a new kidney. Still, I continued my daily routine, praying and talking to God:

> *"If this is the end of my time on earth, I've had a beautiful life,*
> *a terrific family, wonderful friends, and I'm ready to go."*

Meanwhile, doctors had begun testing my youngest daughter, my oldest daughter, and another family member to see if any of them were a match.

On October 21, 2009, while at work, I lost mobility. I continued praying, asking God to guide me safely home. My husband met me in the garage because I couldn't get out of the car. He carried me to the guest room, where I had an out-of-body experience—I was moving toward God and trying to touch His garment.

Then the phone rang.

The message was urgent: *"Hurry to the blood bank. We have an exact match. The doctors want to proceed with the unknown donor kidney—it's younger and they'd prefer not to use one from a family member."*

On October 22, 2009, at the age of 66, I became *anew* at Phoenix Banner University Hospital. It's amazing how God places His angels and people together to do His work. My youngest daughter, a registered nurse, was coming to my aid—and, as God would have it, so was her next-door neighbor, also a registered nurse from the Phoenix Blood Bank. Both of them had to go back on duty to help care for me.

Life continues to be a great blessing. I have lived through three miracles. Trusting and having faith in God is what I treasure most. Always remain in His presence, He can do all things.

ADVICE FOR THOSE WAITING FOR A TRANSPLANT:

- Pray to Almighty God and ask for help. There is nothing He cannot do.

- Be obedient.

- Follow your doctor's instructions and take your medication as prescribed.

- Keep all appointments for your bloodwork.

- Be proactive, ask questions.

Thanks be to God, to my family, to the unknown donor's family who shared a precious organ with me, and to the friends, doctors, and nurses who held my life in their hands. I am forever grateful for God's grace and mercy.

COVID-19 AND MY
KIDNEY TRANSPLANT JOURNEY
Sharon Perry

My name is Sharon Perry, and this is my journey through Chronic Kidney Disease (CKD) and the COVID-19 pandemic.

CKD is a long-term condition where kidney function gradually declines over time. It's often caused by conditions like high blood pressure and diabetes, which damage the kidneys. Other risk factors include heart disease, smoking, and family history. If left untreated, CKD can progress to end-stage renal disease (ESRD), requiring dialysis or a kidney transplant.

During the height of the COVID-19 pandemic, we had to stay six feet apart, wear masks and gloves, and disinfect everything, our homes, cars, clothes, and even ourselves. People were dying, men, women, and children. I remember seeing refrigerated trucks filled with the deceased. It was devastating.

I had been under the care of my nephrologist, Dr. Peter Fumo, for some time. On November 4, 2019, I attended a kidney evaluation at the University of Pennsylvania. By November 19, I had completed a heart echo, treadmill stress test, and given 20 vials of blood. Finally, I was approved and placed on the kidney donor waiting list.

Next, I met with Lydia, the nutritionist, to learn how to eat correctly for my condition. That was the hardest part—I loved meat. I had to learn to read labels, lower my potassium levels, reduce my salt intake (which is in almost everything!), and transition toward a plant-based diet. I was raised eating meat, I'm a carnivore! I hated the changes and became depressed. Nothing I ate seemed right, and my creatinine levels rose. Although I could still urinate, it had bubbles, indicating the presence of protein in the urine.

I applied for disability due to my stage 4 kidney disease, but was denied because I wasn't yet on dialysis. That was a crushing blow.

Depression took over. I lost my sister, Corrie A. Blount. She was my rock. Losing her left me devastated. On top of grieving, I was fighting kidney disease. I fell into denial, drinking, using substances, and smoking Kool cigarettes—all behind closed doors. I was giving up. I didn't know how to save myself. I felt completely alone.

At one point, I visited friends and family to say goodbye. I told them, "This is it. I'm going home to Glory. If I didn't tell you I love you, I'm saying it now."

But God said no. He laid me down to sleep . . . and when I woke up, everything was different. All those desires were gone. To God be the Glory.

Early Sunday morning, May 30, 2021, around 12:30 a.m., I received a call from the University of Pennsylvania. I didn't get to the phone in time, and the call disconnected. I went back to sleep.

Around 7:30 a.m., the phone rang again. A nurse told me I had three potential kidney donors. I was half-asleep and flooded with a mix of emotions: excited, nervous, and overwhelmed. My heart was racing. I was ready to cry, scream, and pray all at once.

That nurse played an important role in my journey. She explained everything despite the challenges of COVID-19. I had already retired early in October 2020 from the Department of Public Welfare to protect myself from the virus. Now, here I was, facing the possibility of a transplant. The nurse, a new mother working from home, was incredibly patient and kind.

I asked what I needed to do—pack a bag? Come to the hospital? She said she'd call back that afternoon with the next steps. I spent the day praying, praising God, and trying to stay calm.

By 4:30 p.m., I couldn't wait any longer. I called the nurse myself. She reassured me that she'd update me soon. At 7:00 p.m., she called, I was third on the list. Then at 8:00 p.m., she called again, I was now first. She told me to pack a bag. I had one hour to get ready and wait for final instructions.

I was pacing in circles, overwhelmed. How would I get there by midnight? Where would I park? But the Holy Spirit told me, "Pack your bags first. Call Uber. Notify everyone once you arrive." So I did just that.

When I arrived, I assumed the surgery would happen immediately. It didn't. My blood pressure was up. I was out of breath. The nurses and staff at Penn had to assess me and complete my chart. Then the nurse said, "Get some rest. Surgery is in the morning." LOL!

Memorial Day, Monday, May 31, 2021. The nurses came in early and said, "Good morning, Ms. Perry. Today is your day."

The staff took me to the OR for a four-hour kidney transplant surgery. I woke up with staples, a catheter, and two drainage holes. I remained in the hospital for 6–7 days and received two rounds of dialysis. Since my donor was deceased, it could take 3–4 weeks for the kidney to start functioning on its own.

I was discharged on Saturday, June 5, 2021. I had to report to the hospital three times a week and undergo regular bloodwork. I also needed dialysis three times a week at a center on Lehigh Avenue. I preferred the later shift; I wasn't moving quickly in the mornings!

The month of June was grueling. I had so many appointments and couldn't drive. I was physically exhausted.

Gradually, the schedule became more manageable. Eventually, I was able to stop dialysis under the care of Dr. Karmic, Dr. Bloom, and Dr. Jordan. But my blood levels were low. I'm anemic. My hemoglobin dropped to 6.5 (normal is around 10), so I had several blood transfusions. Dr. Bloom and Dr. Jordan referred me to Dr. Robert Henry, a hematologist. I began receiving Procrit shots to increase my hemoglobin levels.

On November 5, 2021, my coworkers took me away for a relaxing weekend in Hanover, Maryland. We shopped, laughed, and enjoyed seafood at Crusty Crabs. I returned refreshed.

November 25, 2021, was my first Thanksgiving with my son, Ivan, and his children. I cherished the time with my family.

November 30, 2021, was my six-month transplant anniversary. I gave all glory to God for His mercy and my new kidney.

My recovery has been slow but steady. Nurses and physical therapists visited me weekly during that time. I progressed from a wheelchair to a walker to a cane. Standing for long periods was difficult, but I kept pushing forward.

By January 2022, I was back behind the wheel, driving myself to appointments.

From February to April 2022, I continued monitoring my blood, hemoglobin, and Tacrolimus levels. I received regular Procrit shots and labs to ensure my kidney and blood levels were stable.

On May 31, 2022, I celebrated my first transplant anniversary. Now, in 2025, I've celebrated my fourth Kidneyversary. It's a testament to God's grace and the power of perseverance.

To God be the glory. I'm still here, still standing, still healing. And I'm forever thankful for another chance at life.

"There is no greater love than to lay down one's life for one's friends."
John 15:13 (NLT)

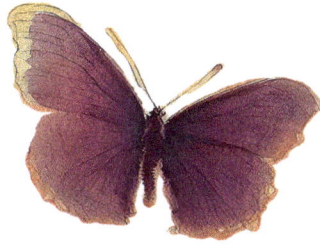

FROM LOVED ONES

I'm Dennis Weaver. I met Yvonne in January 2015, and when we began dating, she told me about everything she was going through with her health. That did not matter to me; I wanted to be with her.

My wife dropped me off at the airport on August 15, 2018, and picked up her sister Sandra at the same time. I was going to Detroit for my birthday, and Sandra came to stay with her while I was gone. Not too long after I landed in Detroit, I received a phone call from Sandra telling me that she had rushed my wife to the hospital. When I talked to my wife, I asked her if she wanted me to turn around and come back. She replied no.

While I was in Detroit, I had a family member to pass, and my wife told me to stay till after the funeral. When I returned home, I went straight to the hospital, and I looked at my wife, and I began to pray. The Lord knows all things, and He does all things well, so I began to pray.

Our son, Lovelle, set up a prayer call, and many people joined from all over the country to pray for my wife. I was at the hospital on the prayer line, and I remember the next morning they called and said they had a Liver.

A few days later, they were taking Yvonne down for surgery, and Angie, Eric, Evangelist Shirley, and I prayed with faith knowing that it was going to be alright. Once she was out of surgery, we were able to see her. She was smiling, laughing, and talking even though she was in a lot of pain.

What I remember the most is when she was able to come home, her wound had not completely healed. She had a hole in her side equal to the size of a big pecan. The nurses showed me how to care for her wound. Even though I had family to help, I guess I didn't want anyone to think I didn't want their help, but they had not been trained. I wasn't selfish, but I wanted to make sure everything was done right. My wife looked up and said, "Let Mattie and Sandra help you."

I remember Yvonne was very weak, but she is a soldier. With her family's help, I am so grateful that God put me in the position to take care of my wife.

Thank you, Jesus, for all you have done.

Yvonne's Husband, Dennis Weaver

When I first heard about my mom's diagnosis, my heart sank. I couldn't believe it was really happening. My first instinct was to pray, and that's exactly what I did—every single day and through every step of her journey. There were moments when doubt tried to creep in, making me wonder if maybe this was her time or if God was calling her home. Still, I held on to faith, knowing how many people were praying for her. Some were close friends and family, and others were people I didn't even know, but they were all standing in prayer with us. With that much faith being lifted, there was no room for doubt.

The night before my mom's transplant, several of us joined a prayer call. Everyone prayed, and afterward, we all went to sleep. Not long after, I got the call that a donor had been found. As I got ready that morning, the emotions hit hard. I cried while thanking and praising God for His miracle.

I have to give credit to my wife, she encouraged me to go see my mom and made the arrangements for me to be there. Neither of us knew her transplant would take place while I was visiting, but God's timing was perfect. Being there to witness her surgery and recovery was powerful. It was living proof of God's strength and faithfulness.

Seeing my mom heal reminded me that God is still in control and still performing miracles. To anyone walking through a situation like this, stay strong and hold on to your faith. God truly is amazing, and His power is real.

Yvonne's son, Eric McMichael

When I first learned about my mom's diagnosis, I felt an overwhelming sense of sadness that this had to happen to her. However, I was raised to believe that God makes no mistakes, so I leaned on the understanding that this situation was in His hands. Being the stoic son, I don't get too high or too low emotionally, so I felt a deep responsibility to stay strong for her.

The waiting period before her transplant was one of the toughest seasons to endure. Watching her health decline and seeing her physically change to the point where she almost didn't look like herself was painful. It was especially difficult because she has always been a giver, someone who loves helping others, and now she was the one in need. Yet, because of who she is, I truly believed it was her time to receive the same love and care she had always given to others.

My faith was never challenged during this time. From the very beginning, I trusted God and left it all on the altar. We were raised to believe in His plan, and I claimed victory on day one.

Being able to stay with her in Arizona, to sit by her side in the hospital, and then witness her make it all the way through to a full recovery was nothing short of miraculous. The experience reminded me how fragile life is, but also how resilient the human spirit can be. Her recovery felt like a gift, another chance at life, and I am deeply grateful that she was blessed to continue her journey of helping others.

To anyone who may be facing a similar struggle, I encourage you not to give up. It's okay to be scared, to cry, to question, and to feel exhausted. But never lose hope. Even in uncertainty, love has a way of carrying us through. Miracles don't always happen suddenly, sometimes they unfold slowly, through quiet moments of prayer and perseverance.

Surround yourself with people who will stand and kneel beside you, and remember that even in your darkest hour, you are not alone. There is a strength within you that you may not even realize you have yet.

Yvonne's son,
Shariff McMichael

When I first learned about the severity of my mother's diagnosis, I was in shock. She had endured sickness before and had already conquered cancer, so to hear that she was now in complete liver failure felt like a point of no return. My first thought was, "Lord, how much more can she bear?"

The Bible tells us, "*In this world you will have trouble. But take heart! I have overcome the world.*" John 16:33 (NIV)

In that moment, I struggled to hold onto that truth because all I could see was the possibility of losing my mom.

During the waiting season before her transplant, I coped by diving headfirst into caregiving. It became my way of fighting fear. I didn't want to regret it if she didn't make it.

Scripture reminds us, "*Whatever you do, work at it with all your heart, as working for the Lord.*" Colossians 3:23 (NIV)

Caring for my mother was not only an act of love, it was an act of worship. I wanted to be sure I had done everything humanly possible to give her the best chance at life, and in doing so, I found peace even in the face of uncertainty.

But truthfully, my faith was shaken. As a pastor, I wrestled with hard questions: Why would a woman who had dedicated her life to God, a faithful servant, be stricken with such a terminal illness? In those moments, I found myself echoing the psalmist's cry: "*How long, Lord? Will you forget me forever?*" Psalm 13:1 (NIV) Yet even in doubt, I turned to praise and worship. Like Paul and Silas, who prayed and sang hymns while locked in prison (Acts 16:25), I found that worship unlocked peace in the darkest nights. It didn't erase the pain, but it reminded me of God's presence.

When my mother survived and recovered, I realized it was not just an answer to prayer, but a miracle in the making. The true miracle wasn't just the transplant—it was that God had sustained her for twenty-plus years with a disease that could have taken her life long before. Scripture says, "*The Lord sustains them on their sickbed and restores them from their bed of illness.*" Psalm 41:3 (NIV) That verse became real to me as I watched my mother's life be spared time and time again until the day came for her healing breakthrough.

To anyone reading this who may be facing a similar struggle, let me encourage you: the outcome may not always look like my mother's, but God is still faithful. "*We walk by faith, not by sight.*" 2 Corinthians 5:7 (KJV) Sometimes the healing comes through a miracle, and sometimes the miracle is the strength to endure. As Romans 5:3-4 reminds us, "*We glory in tribulations also: knowing that tribulation worketh patience; and patience, experience; and experience, hope.*"

Good things happen to bad people, and bad things happen to good people, but no matter what, keep the faith. Live with no regrets. Stay pure with God and stay close to your family. Above all, remember: "*Those who hope in the Lord will renew their strength. They will soar on wings like eagles; they will run and not grow weary, they will walk and not faint.*" Isaiah 40:41 (NIV)

My mother's journey has shown me that miracles come in many forms. Sometimes the greatest miracle is not the healing itself, but the strength God gives us to persevere until His promises are revealed.

Yvonne's son,
Lovelle Mc Michael

Upon my arrival in Arizona on August 15, 2018, I was immediately struck by Yvonne's appearance. As we embraced, I couldn't help but express my concern, "I don't like how you look." She reassured me that she was fine, just a little tired, and asked me to drive.

Once we got to the apartment, the first thing she did was sit down and, after catching her breath, went into the bedroom and lay down. I was observing her the whole time, and I did not feel comfortable, so I called 911. They came, and because they knew her history, they advised us to go to the emergency room after testing, and they admitted her to the hospital.

It was good that we came because things had changed dramatically. I called Angie and Lovelle because they knew more about her history than I did. Aunt Yvonne came because I was upset, not knowing enough about her history.

During the two weeks I was there, Yvonne was placed on an emergency list for a liver transplant. Despite the uncertainty, she maintained a smile, unwavering in her trust in God.

People used to call us "salt and pepper" due to our contrasting complexions. I was darker, and she was lighter. Now, Yvonne was my complexion, but it was incredible to see how her complexion had changed, a testament to her resilience.

Day after day, I went to sit with her to make sure everything was okay and was running smoothly with the doctors and with her care. To God be the glory. I had to pull back tears because I was so blessed that she was still here, because I didn't want both of us crying at the same time.

She had a liver transplant, and it was a success. After the second week, they showed me how to clean her wounds, but her loving husband wanted to change her bandages himself. I was there to help with whatever and wherever they needed me.

God is good, and my faith was strengthened by witnessing my sister's unwavering focus on Jesus. Seven years later, we continue to celebrate the miraculous healing power of God, working through the doctors and nurses He anointed to care for her.

Yvonne's sister,
Sandra Merrill

Over the years, my sister has experienced several health challenges through which by God's grace, she has overcome them. When I received the news of her liver failure, I was undoubtedly shocked, but by God's grace, my emotions remained stabilized.

I had many thoughts and asked some questions for gaining a better understanding of the seriousness of her illness but remained prayerful that God's will would be done in her life. During this time, I was able to lean on the unwavering support and prayers of a godly mother and sisters in the faith. The word of God promises us in James 5:16 that the prayer of a righteous man has great power to prevail.

I remember talking with my sister one night while she was in the hospital awaiting a decision on a liver transplant and she mentioned feeling death and darkness hovering over her room. I remember encouraging her through God's word in what He promised us through His servant Paul that whatever is true, whatever is honorable, whatever is right, whatever is pure, whatever is lovely, whatever is of good repute, if there is any excellence and if anything worthy of praise, dwell on these things (Philippians 4:8). It is only the word of God that will bring life to those who receive it.

As human beings, we seek to support in tangible ways and feel helpless when our physical abilities are inadequate. This emotion was amplified for me, as my sister and I reside in different states. During this time by God's grace, my niece Angie had established an Amazon account for allowing people from all over the country to contribute to my sister's necessities. In addition to meeting her physical needs, the Lord permitted me to create a keepsake book with pages of His promises for reminding my sister of His faithfulness during times of fear, doubt, and distress.

Thank the Lord for His mercy, compassion, grace, and abounding lovingkindness towards my sister in keeping her here to this day! The Lord promises us in Psalm 138:8 that He will accomplish what concerns me; Your lovingkindness, O LORD, is everlasting; Do not forsake the works of Your hands.

I praise the Lord for allowing many to see the work of the Lord's hands in my sister's life! The Bible speaks about how many believed in Jesus because of the miracles He performed. It is my hope and prayer that the miracle seen in my sister's life by the hand of the Lord will not be a fleeting moment, but one that will bring about conviction of sin leading to repentance, faith, and trust in the one, true, and living God who is able to not just heal the physical body, but also able to save the soul.

Yvonne's sister,
Bianca

WHAT A TROOPER!

All the thoughts and feelings I have when I reflect on the miracle of my sister's life. Tootsie, affectionately known as Yvonne, has called me her Big Little Brother since I can remember.

It was like she never let you know she was going through a health crisis. She kept the faith and believed God every step of the way. As my big sister, she let me see her going through, depending on Him, despite the illness she was experiencing. That's what a trooper does: they keep doing the job they have been trained to do, regardless of the weather, the conditions, or the time of day.

You are never trained to overcome difficulties until you experience difficulties. Toot's trusting Jesus made it possible to see her overcome (recover) when the doctors said differently, and God's timing is based on faith in Him when the odds are against you.

So, illness never prevented her from being there for those that needed her; it was more of me looking on than for my experiencing it. Momma Toot's is who she was to everyone, and she continued to be and do for everyone while she went through her adversity.

It was by God's grace and His mercy that allowed her to keep it all together. If it weren't for the picture of her in the hospital, you would not know or even believe that she was at that point in her life. His favor in the transplant was the miracle that never ended; the step-by-step acceptance, recovery, and now the renewed life living are what make the trooper do what they continue to do.

I am grateful for the testimony she can now share because she allowed God to work on her and bring her out to tell the story of Jesus' amazing grace. To God be the glory for all He has done, and I know Yvonne will continue to speak of His goodness that will encourage and inspire others to keep the faith and be a witness of the love the Father has for his dear children!

If He did it for Toots, I know He will do it for those who hear her story, trust God, and give Him their all, as she has.

Yvonne's brother,
Curtis

Unshakeable faith, that's what comes to my mind when I think of her experience during her time of struggle before the transplant. When I talked to her on the phone, I knew that it was time for me to be there. I made travel arrangements the same day and was there before nightfall.

When I saw her in the condition she was in with the swelling, I knew it was serious. The nurses would come and drain the fluid, and before the day was done, the nurses had to do it again.

Always remembering God's faithfulness and how he has brought us all through so many difficulties, and knowing how strong her faith was, there was no fear.

We knew we had to trust God and wait on Him. We stand on the shoulders of a woman of faith, Emma Schley, her grandmother, my mother. Her faith never wavered, and we watched how she went through difficulties, never complaining, just staying focused on God. Tootsie, as we affectionately call (Yvonne Weaver), possesses those same qualities. We are eternally grateful for the example Tootsie set before us.

Aunt Yvonne

When I first learned of Yvonne's diagnosis, I was nervous and fearful—but also hopeful. I was so impressed by the way she endured the long waiting season before her transplant. Her faith carried her through, even when it was tested, and I found myself praying, praying, and praying some more—believing God for victory.

Watching Yvonne survive and recover meant everything to me. It was truly witnessing God's miracle in real time, and my faith was strengthened in the process.

To anyone reading this who may be facing similar struggles, I want to encourage you: when life feels out of your control, lean into prayer.

Trust God, read His Word, and believe that He can work it out on your behalf. No matter the circumstance, He has everything under control.

Mattie Williams, Yvonne's Spiritual Sister and Longtime Friend

*"I will give you a new heart
and put a new spirit in you."*
Ezekiel 36:26 (NIV)

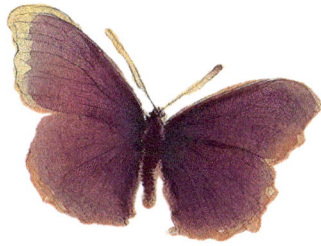

EPILOGUE

An epilogue often marks the end of a journey, but in reality, my journey is far from over.

Surviving a liver transplant was not the end of my story. It was simply the beginning of a new chapter. Every day I wake up, I am reminded that this life is a gift, one that I do not take for granted. I strive to live my best life, to walk in my purpose, and to be a blessing to others.

There are moments when the weight of what I have endured settles on me, and I think back to the hard days, the pain, the uncertainty, the countless hospital stays. But rather than dwell on those hardships, I choose to focus on the joy that has come from this journey.

"For the joy of the Lord is my strength."

Nehemiah 8:10

That joy is what sustains me. That joy is what pushes me forward.

The transplant may have saved my life, but the journey never truly ends. Not a single day goes by that I don't thank God for His mercy and grace. I also pray for the medical teams that took care of me, for my donor's family, and for every person who supported me along the way.

Being a survivor means that I must continue to fight for my health. I have a responsibility to myself, to my family, and to the people who still need to hear my testimony.

Each day, I:

- Take my anti-rejection medication so that my body continues to accept this precious gift of life.

- Eat healthy and make wise choices to ensure my body remains strong.

- Stay active, even on the days when I don't feel 100 percent.

- Encourage others who are still in the fight, reminding them that miracles are real.

I don't know what tomorrow holds, none of us do. What I do know is that I have been given another chance, and I refuse to waste it.

> *"This is the day which the Lord hath made; we will rejoice and be glad in it."*
>
> Psalm 118:24

If there is one thing I want you to take from this book, it is this:

God is still in the miracle-working business. I am not here because of my own strength. I am here because of His.

Through every hardship, every setback, and every moment of uncertainty, God was with me. He never left me. And if you are facing your own battle, whether it be illness, loss, or any challenge that feels impossible, know that He is with you, too.

I am living proof that there is nothing too hard for God.

I pray that my story has encouraged you to hold onto faith, hope, and perseverance. No matter what you are facing, remember:

You are stronger than you think. You are not alone. And your story is far from over.

I am a walking, talking miracle—and so are you.

"Remember His marvelous works which He has done."
I Chronicles 16:12 (NKJV)

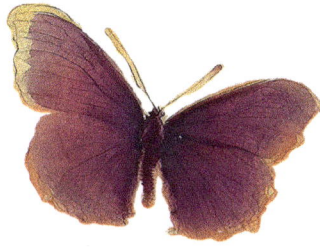

ACKNOWLEDGMENT

To my beloved husband, Dennis, and my three sons, Eric, Shariff, and Lovelle, you are my greatest blessings. As young teenagers, you witnessed a transformation in my life when God showed me the path I needed to take. I chose to live for Him, to be a godly mother, and to set an example for you, so that one day, you would know the kind of woman worthy of becoming your wife.

> *"He who finds a wife finds a good thing and obtains favor from the Lord."*
>
> Proverbs 18:22

To my daughters-in-love and my precious grandchildren, your love and support have been a source of joy and strength. I especially express gratitude to Dr. Angie Williams-McMichael, my personal doctor and daughter-in-love, who walked beside me through my illness, and to her right-hand girl, Fredreka Graham, your dedication means more than words can convey.

To my father, who went home to be with the Lord in January 2023, and his loving wife, thank you for every prayer lifted and every call made to check on me. To my Aunt Yvonne, my sisters Sandra Merrill and Bianca Cummings, and my brother Curtis T. Schley and his wife Patricia, your presence and care were a comfort beyond measure.

To my sisters in Christ, Mattie Williams, Shirley Lewis, and Lynn Young, who stepped in and cared for me, and to my dear friend Pauline Sims, who was by my side from the very beginning of this journey in 1995–96—your unwavering support has been a gift.

To my Pastor Joyce Jay and my Worship Life Center Family—your prayers and visits lifted my spirit. To my Five-Fold Ministry friends across Arizona, Philadelphia, and worldwide, your calls, visits, and encouragement reminded me that I was never alone.

Finally, to every person who sent a care package, a card, a monetary gift, or simply whispered a prayer on my behalf—your kindness has left an indelible mark on my heart. I am eternally grateful.

ACKNOWLEDGMENT

I am here today as a *Walking, Talking Miracle*, not just because of my own faith but because of the love, prayers, and sacrifices of each of you. May God bless you abundantly and draw you ever closer to Him.

With a heart full of gratitude,

Yvonne

"Though outwardly we are wasting away, yet inwardly we are being renewed day by day."
2 Corinthians 4:16 (NIV)

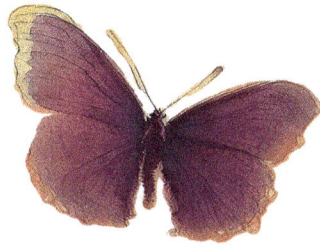

ABOUT THE AUTHOR

As a native of Philadelphia, Evangelist Yvonne Weaver was trained in missions, administration, and evangelism under the leadership of Dr. Marlene Talley of Christian Youth Rally and Faith Hope & Love C.O.G.I.C. Pastor John H. Roberts. She has also served under the leadership of Pastor Curtis T. Schley of Life Changing Word C.O.G.I.C. in Abington, Pennsylvania.

Evangelist Weaver's experiences have afforded her the opportunity to work in the following ministries: prayer & intercession, deliverance, prison, and new members. Her ministry extends into the foreign field— The Chez Republic, where she served as a missionary witnessing to lost souls. Matthew 25:35-40.

God transitioned Evangelist Weaver to Phoenix, Arizona, in 2004 to serve Impacted for Purpose Ministries under the leadership of Pastor Lovelle McMichael in the following capacities: Director of Ministry Outreach and Intercession. Her signature messages include: "You Are Only a Thought Away from God's Presence" and "God said, Trust Me."

SCRIPTURES EVANGELIST WEAVER LIVE BY:

"But Jesus beheld them, and said unto them, with men this is impossible; but with God all things are possible."

Matthew 19:26

"Death and life are in the power of the tongue: and they that love it shall eat the fruit thereof. "

Proverbs 18:21

"It is the spirit that quickeneth; the flesh profiteth nothing: the words that I speak unto you, are spirit, and they are life."

John 6:63

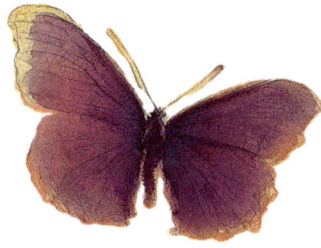

ABOUT LIVER TRANSPLANTATION AND AFRICAN AMERICANS

A LEGACY OF HOPE AND INEQUALITY

Introduction

Organ transplantation is one of medicine's greatest triumphs. For families who have witnessed a loved one return from the edge of death, the experience feels nothing short of miraculous.

But miracles have not always been shared equally.

African Americans have long faced barriers in access to liver transplantation—barriers built not from biology, but from social inequities, systemic exclusion, and historic medical mistrust. Understanding this history honors not only the miracle of Yvonne's survival but also the resilience of many others whose stories are rarely told.

A BRIEF HISTORY OF LIVER TRANSPLANTATION

Early Breakthroughs (1960s–1970s)

- **1967:** Dr. Thomas Starzl performs the first successful human liver transplant.
- Procedures remain experimental, costly, and geographically limited.
- African Americans face systemic exclusion from specialty hospitals and are rarely referred for advanced procedures.

Progress Expands (1980s–1990s)

Key national reforms begin to expand fairness:

- **1984:** National Organ Transplant Act
- **UNOS** established to manage nationwide waiting lists
- Standardized criteria improves evaluation and listing processes

Yet disparities persisted, driven by:

- Insurance and financial barriers
- Later referrals for evaluation
- Mistrust rooted in historic medical injustices
- Higher incidence of liver diseases in Black communities

The Modern Era (2000s–Present)

Liver transplantation is now a standard treatment for end-stage liver disease. Still:

- African Americans make up 13% of the U.S. population, but a disproportionate share of those needing transplants
- They wait longer for organs—sometimes despite equal urgency
- Post-transplant outcomes are poorer due to social determinants of health:
  - Income
  - Housing stability
  - Transportation
  - Access to specialists
  - Structural bias

These disparities are not biological—they are social.

Global and National Context

In 2023:

- **103,000+** people were on the national transplant waiting list
- Every **9 minutes** someone is added
- **17 people die each day** waiting
- Over **46,000** transplants were performed
- One donor can save **up to 8 lives**

Globally, the need for organs far exceeds availability. Despite this, advances in science—stem cells, regenerative medicine, 3D bioprinting—continue to offer emerging hope.

WHY THIS MATTERS FOR AFRICAN AMERICAN COMMUNITIES

For African Americans, every successful transplant is:

- A **medical victory**
- A **social victory**
- A **spiritual victory**

It represents overcoming barriers, bias, history, and inequity.

Yvonne's survival is more than her personal triumph—it is a symbol of what is possible when advocacy, persistence, and faith meet opportunity.

HOW YOU CAN HELP

1. **Become an Organ Donor**

   Register at www.organdonor.gov and inform your family.

2. **Support Equity in Healthcare**

   Advocacy improves access, education, and outcomes.

3. **Share Stories that Inspire Change**

   Stories like Yvonne's remind the world that inequality is real—and so is hope.

FINAL REFLECTION

The story of liver transplantation is one of science, perseverance, and grace. But it is also a story of inequity—one that we must continue to confront.

May Evangelist Yvonne Weaver's journey inspire others to believe, to support, and to fight for a future where every person has an equal chance at life.

www.ingramcontent.com/pod-product-compliance
Lightning Source LLC
Chambersburg PA
CBHW052118030426
42335CB00025B/3039